I0766695

LIFE, HOPE, AND HEALING...
SURVIVING A CANCER DIAGNOSIS

GWENDOLYN W. BURRELL

LIFE, HOPE, AND HEALING...
SURVIVING A CANCER DIAGNOSIS

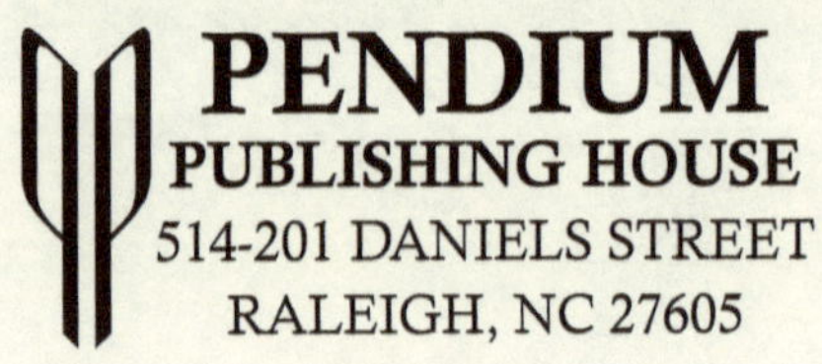

PENDIUM
PUBLISHING HOUSE
514-201 DANIELS STREET
RALEIGH, NC 27605

For information, please visit our Website at
www.pendiumpublishing.com

PENDIUM Publishing and its logo
are registered trademarks.

LIFE, HOPE, and HEALING…
Surviving a Cancer Diagnosis
By Gwendolyn W. Burrell

Copyright © Gwendolyn W. Burrell, 2015
All Rights Reserved.

ISBN: 978-1-936513-36-9

PUBLISHER'S NOTE

Without limiting the rights under the copyright reserved above, no
part of this publication may be reproduced, stored in or introduced
into a retrieval system, or transmitted, in any form, or by any means
(electronic, mechanical, photocopying, recording, or otherwise),
without the prior written permission of both the copyright owner and
the above publisher of this book.

Unless otherwise noted, Scripture quotations are taken from the Holy
Bible, New International Version.

If you purchased this book without a cover you should be aware that
the book is stolen property. It was reported as "unsold and destroyed"
to the publisher and neither the author nor the publisher has received
any payment for this "stripped book."

This book is printed on acid-free paper.

DEDICATION

This book is dedicated to my husband, Gary, my sons, Jordan and Gordan, my father, Richard, Jr., my sisters, Patricia, Eleanor, and Carolyn, my brother, Richard, III, my daughter-in-law, Meagan, my nieces, nephews, my brother-in-law, William, my mother-in-law, Bernice, and dear friends who all supported me through words of encouragement, prayer, presence, preparing or purchasing meals, or traveling with me to medical appointments and staying with me through surgery and recovery.

I also dedicate this book to my Pastor J. Jasper Wilkins, Jr., First Lady Cheryl Wilkins, Deacon James Ragland, Sr, Deacon and Mrs. Leon Harris, and all other Deacons and Wives, Minister Latangela Hyman, Elder Jackie Jeter, and Elder Mischella McQueen, all of Wake Chapel Church, Raleigh, North Carolina, who laid hands on me, prayed fervently for me, prophesied to me and encouraged me throughout this journey. As well as other members of my church family, who were very supportive. The number is too great to mention individually.

Lastly, throughout the writing of this book, I remembered my mother, Vivian Waddell, whose strength and tenacity I will always remember; her examples I follow daily.

FOREWORD

This book is not a foreboding tale of woe. It is however a wonderful story of Gwen's courage, tenacity and strong faith. Gwen clearly articulates the plethora of emotions and stages that confronts a person who is diagnosed with cancer. This story is simply amazing in that she talks specifically as it relates to her bout with a stage 4 extremely rare form of cancer but generally she suggests how you can really overcome any struggle in life. The victory is gained by properly utilizing your faith as an antidote. This antidote produces for you a change in your thinking as well as provides a quantum leap in motivation. Definitely the combination of faith and proper treatment provided a cure that caused her to author this book which by the way is a guide to help promote health and wellness in all areas of life.

J. Jasper Wilkins, Jr. Senior Pastor of Wake Chapel Church (WCC) Raleigh, North Carolina

CONTENTS

Preface 11

Chapter One: The Dreaded Diagnosis 13

Chapter Two: Seeking God and Listening
                 To His Voice 21

Chapter Three: Moving To The Next Phase...
                 Preparing For Battle 24

Chapter Four: Following God's Advice 36

Chapter Five: Giving God the Glory 40

Chapter Six: You Don't Look Sick 46

Chapter Seven: Caregivers... The Faith of Those
                 around You 49

Chapter Eight: Resources 52

PREFACE

*Dear friend, I pray that you may enjoy good
health and that all may go well with you, even
as your soul is getting along well.*
3 John 1:2 NIV

I write this book because I know the feeling of hearing the words "It is cancer." Whether it is you who has received the diagnosis, a family member, friend, or co-worker, the news can be devastating! Immediately, everyone thinks of the worst outcome. Hopefully this book will change that thought pattern! Think Life, Hope, and Healing! I did, and today, one year after the diagnosis of stage four neuroendocrine cancer, I have been healed by My Almighty God! God has no respect of persons, just like he healed me, he can also heal you! Through this book, I will share my journey from diagnosis to healing! I pray that it is a blessing to you!

> *Dear God, I come humbly before you this day.
> Lord I know you to be the great physician, my
> healer. Lord there are many others who are
> dealing with having been diagnosed with cancer.
> We know that you are bigger than cancer. I
> pray that you will touch each patient reading
> this book, each family member, caregiver, and*

friend that they will be encouraged to seek you and rely on you as they seek treatment and care. We stand on your word that says, "By your stripes, we were healed." I pray this prayer in the precious name of Jesus. Amen

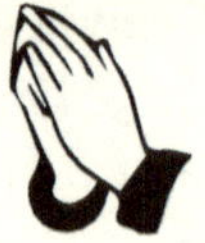

CHAPTER ONE

The Dreaded Diagnosis

What do you do when the unexpected happens? Trust God! The fall of September, 2013 was an awakening for me of the true lack of control that we as human beings have over our lives and life's circumstances. On the eve of September 23, 2013, I began having excruciating pain in my abdominal area. I had experienced this numerous times during the preceding three years. Visits to emergency rooms resulted in CT Scans, ultrasounds, and IV pain medicines, but the diagnosis was always inconclusive. I was told it could be gas, stress induced symptoms, gastritis, or indigestion. The diagnosis from each visit was usually something different, but the overall theme was "we cannot find anything wrong." I would go home, sleep off the pain meds and the symptoms would subside. But in September 2013, I knew something was wrong; this time in addition to the pain, I was vomiting violently. I called the on call physician at my primary care physician's office. She suggested going to the emergency room or if I could, wait until morning and see my Gastroenterologist. I knew the emergency room routine and did not feel like waiting hours for yet another inconclusive diagnosis and a two hundred dollar bill! I took a couple of pain pills from a previous visit, medicine for nausea, and medicine for gas, since I was previously told it could just be gas. The next morning I awoke feeling a little better, but still in some pain. I called my Gastroenterologist's office to make an appointment. Although, she had no availability, her assistant asked me to come in since the office was just opening and she would fit me in. That was welcoming news. I got dressed and drove myself to her office.

Once I arrived at her office, and she entered the examination room, she saw the look of pain and discomfort. She indicated that we needed to get to the bottom of what was going on. We discussed the recurring episodes over the last few years.

A month prior to this visit, I had arthroscopic knee surgery to repair a torn meniscus and had been taking an anti-inflammatory medicine for quite some time. The doctor indicated that this time could be an ulcer from the anti-inflammatory medicine or a problem with my gallbladder. She ordered an Ultrasound. I left her office for the radiology center. The technician at the radiology center was extremely kind and enjoyed her work. We talked throughout the ultrasound about various topics. The one thing that was obvious about her was that she was a Christian. She was very thorough, more so than any technicians who had administered ultrasounds in the emergency rooms I had visited. I noticed that she repeatedly scanned one area, and then thoroughly scanned other areas of my abdominal region and side. When I arose from the table, I had an idea that there would be some resolution from her detailed work.

As I was driving home, I received a telephone call from my Gastroenterologist's office. Her assistant indicated that the doctor received the results of the ultrasound and she wanted to know if I could be at her office the next morning at 8:30 to discuss the results. I said yes, and hung up. There was no urgency in her voice so I thought to myself, it must be an ulcer. I drove home and told my husband, Gary, of the appointment.

At 8:30 the next morning, we arrived and were escorted to an examination room. The doctor entered, but was not her jovial self. She had a look of concern on her face as she spoke to us. She indicated that the ultrasound revealed a mass in my mesenteric area and lesions on my liver which appeared as if it could be cancer that had spread to my liver. She scheduled me for a CT scan and asked that I do that after leaving her office. I was stunned, that was not what I expected to hear! Although the news was stunning, I had peace. I am a very inquisitive person, but I couldn't even ask questions at that point.

Gary and I proceeded to the radiology center. The ride was quiet as we were both processing what we had just heard. Upon arrival, I checked in. I noticed a separate mammogram section and thought, oh well; I may as well get a mammogram also since it had been over a year since my last one. I was able to have a mammogram screening while waiting for the CT. Shortly after returning to the waiting room, I was called back for the CT. The CT took about 45 minutes; my upper and lower abdominal areas were scanned.

That afternoon, I received a telephone call from my

Gastroenterologist. She advised me that she received the CT results and she contacted an oncologist for me to follow up with. She indicated someone from his office would be calling me to schedule an appointment. That afternoon I received a telephone call scheduling the appointment for the next day. I was told to pick up a copy of the radiology report and CD. I picked them up. As soon as I returned to my car, I opened the report to read it. Being a former premed major, I was familiar with many of the medical terms. Those I was unfamiliar with, I googled on my iPhone. The report indicated that there was a nodule on my small intestines, a mass in the mesenteric area and eight lesions on my liver indicative of "carcinoid cancer" with liver metastases.

Really, some type of cancer? I had never heard of that type of cancer. My research indicated that carcinoid tumors are a rare, slow growing cancer that is difficult to diagnose. I sat there in my car and cried. How could that be possible? I was in great shape, felt great most days, was going to the gym consistently, had never had any serious illnesses, not even a cavity, at the age of 51 years old, and knew of no history of cancer in my family. I pulled myself together, returned the report to the envelope and drove home.

Once I arrived home, my research began. I read many articles and visited specific websites pertaining to carcinoid and neuroendocrine cancer, the two names are used interchangeably. I found that carcinoid tumors are a type of neuroendocrine tumor, which means that they come from the cells of the nervous and endocrine system, and can produce hormones, such as histamine and serotonin. The tumors can be found in primary sites such as the colon, intestines, pancreas, or lungs. Gastrointestinal carcinoid tumors can cause symptoms such as abdominal pain, constipation, and cramping. Some people experience "Carcinoid Syndrome." The symptoms of Carcinoid Syndrome include diarrhea, flushing of the skin, wheezing, and shortness of breath, abdominal cramps, and heart palpitations. Cramping was the only symptom I experienced over the years. Because the symptoms can be vague, and this cancer is so rare, doctors do not think of it. Some are not even aware of it!

My husband, Gary and I went to the appointment with the oncologist. He reviewed the scans with us and the radiology report after taking some initial history. He indicated that he suspected neuroendocrine cancer, which was a rare cancer of the neuroendocrine system. The origin was unknown and the cause of this type of cancer is unknown. He ordered bloodwork and a liver biopsy. The liver biopsy was scheduled several days later at Rex Hospital in Raleigh. Although I had researched liver biopsy and knew what would take place, I was extremely nervous. However, the staff was very kind and did an outstanding job reassuring me and taking great care of me. The nurses wished me well after the procedure. Two days later, on October 1, 2013, I returned to see the oncologist. He confirmed that it was neuroendocrine cancer, which is a rare slow growing cancer. The biopsy revealed that it was grade 2, meaning it wasn't the slowest growing, but wasn't aggressive. As the oncologist was speaking, I heard him state that it was stage 4 neuroendocrine cancer. A very rare slow growing cancer that had spread from an unknown primary, meaning he didn't know where the cancer originated, to the mesenteric area, membranous tissue that attaches to the intestinal tract, and to my liver. While he was speaking, I also heard the voice of God saying, it's okay, all is well, you are healed!

Hearing the voice of God say to me it was well and I was healed was a source of comfort and peace. That was the message that gave me hope throughout my journey! I knew I would stand on the promises of God!

Scripture Confirmation:

"For I know the plans I have for you," declares the Lord, "plans to prosper you and not to harm you, plans to give you hope and a future."
Jeremiah 29:11 NIV

The oncologist indicated that he had only seen two or three cases in his career, but he would do all he could for me.

My next thought, was my family. My husband Gary was with me, but I had to tell my sons, my father and my siblings. I knew the news would be devastating and I did not want them to be sad. My son Jordan was getting married in three months and I did not want to put a damper on his joy and that of my now daughter, Meagan. But, Jordan called first and I shared everything with him. I then told my sisters, who told my father, brother, nephews, and nieces.

As I expected, the news was difficult to bear. I struggled with how to tell my youngest son, Gordan, who was a senior in high school. I did not want to ruin his senior year or have him worried about me. Initially, I told him it was a tumor that was found and I would have to have some medical treatment. I explained what a tumor was. As days passed,

I didn't feel right not giving Gordan complete information. It wasn't fair that others knew and I had only provided him with some of the truth. Later, I explained to him that it was a slow growing cancer. I assured him that I was seeking the best treatment and I would be fine. I reiterated to each of my family members that I was okay and I had to simply gear up for battle. However, I was confident that God was with me.

Scripture Confirmation:

> *Let us then approach God's throne of grace with confidence, so that we may receive mercy and find grace to help us in our time of need.* **Hebrews 4:16 NIV**

None of us expect to hear that we have been diagnosed with cancer. I know I didn't. I did not know of anyone in my family who had ever had cancer, so I was under the impression that I did not have to be concerned about that illness. I later found out that my paternal grandfather had colon cancer. Through it all and through any situation where we have no control, we must trust God!

Scripture Confirmation:

> *Trust in the Lord with all your heart and lean not on your own understanding; in all your ways submit to him, and he will make your paths straight.* **Proverbs 3: 5 6 NIV**

> *But blessed is the one who trust in the Lord, whose confidence is in him. They will be like a*

tree planted by the water that sends out its roots by the stream. It does not fear when heat comes; its leaves are always green. It has no worries in a year of drought and never fails to bear fruit.
Jeremiah 17: 7-8 NIV

CHAPTER TWO

Seeking God and Listening To His Voice

I have always been in tuned to God's voice. I recall the day I graduated from law school. Before graduation, I was reflecting on the last four years of working full time, taking care of my son Jordan, and going to law school classes at night, studying, writing papers, exams, and studying for and passing the Bar Exam. For the first time, I thought about all I had endured and I had made it through! God spoke to me in my spirit and brought to mind the scripture, Matthew 6:33 "But seek first the kingdom of God and His righteousness, and, all these things shall be added to you." I knew from that moment that as long as I kept my focus on God and sought Him, he would take care of everything else.

One day I was driving on Interstate 40 in the right lane; there were no vehicles in front of me and I was cruising at a decent speed. I heard God say "move into the left lane." I did not see any reason to do so, but I did. As I traveled another mile or so, a vehicle sped off the exit ramp and crashed into the vehicle in the right travel lane. I was in awe. I thanked God for his protection! I can share many examples of the benefits I have received over the years, all because, I listened to God's voice and I obeyed. Let me share one more occasion with you.

Once I was diagnosed with neuroendocrine cancer, the first oncologist I visited wanted me to begin an aggressive schedule of chemotherapy the next week. His plan was for me to have chemotherapy five days then take three days off over the course of four weeks. He had his nurse call and make an appointment to have a port inserted in my chest the following day. Things were moving very swiftly. As my husband and I left his office, I received a telephone call from my primary care physician, who had been notified of the diagnosis. He called to apologize for what I was dealing with and to let me know he would be researching specialists that I could see, because it is such a rare cancer. I advised him of the appointment to put in a port. He said in his opinion, I may as well do it because regardless of who I saw, they would probably want that done. I wasn't sure as I did not feel strongly about having that done and neither did Gary.

When we arrived home, I continued my research on neuroendocrine tumors and treatment. All medical journal articles I read indicated that chemotherapy was generally not effective on neuroendocrine tumors. That night Gary and I discussed this. He did not have a good feeling about me getting the port put in and neither did I. The next morning, I clearly heard God's voice say cancel the appointment. I called the hospital and cancelled the procedure. I was asked if I wanted to reschedule the procedure, I said no.

The next morning, I was just about to leave for work. I received a telephone call from the oncologist. He asked how I was feeling then proceeded to tell me that he took my case to a tumor conference the previous day and his colleagues did a case study of my medical records over the last five years. He said they agreed that chemotherapy was not the best course of treatment for the type of cancer I had been diagnosed with. He asked when I was scheduled to get the port put in. I told him I was scheduled the previous day; however, I did not go. He asked why. I told him God told me not to. He politely said, "I'm glad you listened to God and not me." This was confirmation that I would continue to seek God and listen for his direction as we navigated this trial. This enhanced my faith. I knew for sure that God was with me and was going to get me through this. I reflected on the words He spoke to me in the oncologist's office, "it's okay, all is well, you are healed!"

Scripture Confirmation:

> *For the Lord will be at your side and will keep your foot from being snared.* **Proverbs 3:26 NIV**

CHAPTER THREE

Moving To The Next Phase…
Preparing For Battle

The oncologist said, let's schedule an appointment so that you can come in and we discuss next steps. I said to him, "I appreciate what you have done, but I have to find an oncologist who has experience with this type of cancer." He said "I understand; if there is anything I can do for you, let me know." I said "okay," and our conversation ended.

I returned to my research to find a local oncologist who specialized in Neuroendocrine Cancer. I visited the Carcinoid Cancer Foundation website. The website contained a listing by state of physicians with knowledge of the disease and those who were considered specialists.

Whatever condition you are dealing with, research related organizations and foundations where you can obtain information about your condition, specialists, treatments, and services. You will be more informed and empowered; you can have a thorough knowledge and understanding of your condition, and actively participate in your care.

I found a local oncologist on the site, called the office and scheduled an appointment to see him. I completed a medical authorization so that he could obtain copies of my medical records, biopsy tissue, results, and scans.

My husband Gary, and my sisters, Eleanor, Patricia, and Carolyn accompanied me to my appointment. My sisters had traveled two hours to be with me. When I opened the door they all stared at me, then Patricia, my oldest sister said, "You look good; you're doing better than we are!" Once I told my family of the diagnosis, everyone was shocked and the news was very upsetting. Having not seen me in a while, they did not know what to expect. Many of my friends and family members later expressed that they were apprehensive about talking to me or seeing me because they did not know what to say, how I was handling the news, or what I looked like. They were used to seeing me vibrant and healthy and did not want to think about me looking "sickly!" God was keeping me! He was keeping my mind strong and keeping me in a state of good health and strong.

At the appointment, I found the oncologist more knowledgeable of neuroendocrine cancer. We discussed the disease and its varied course. It is a very different cancer that affects people in different ways. What one person may experience may be completely different from what another person may experience. I found this to be true, because I never had any of the symptoms, other than abdominal cramping.

He recommended that I begin treatment that would consist of monthly injections of a drug by the name of

Sandostatin. This drug was known to shrink tumors and stop the growth of the tumors. Sandostatin is administered in dosages of 10mg, 20mg, 30mg, and 40mg. He suggested that I begin with a dosage of 30 mg. I inquired about surgery. During my research, I found that surgery was the best course of action for the best outcome, and possible cure. He indicated that he would meet with his surgical team; however, because of the location of the mesenteric tumor and the number of tumors in my liver, he did not consider me to be a surgical candidate.

At the conclusion of the appointment, the oncologist printed a copy of the visit notes for me. The visit notes included about 3 pages of research notes, and mortality rates. I wasn't interested in mortality rates, because no one can date stamp me! My sister Eleanor must have noticed a change in my expression as I read the information. She has to know everything, so she asked me for the documents. As she begin to read the information, I told her not to focus on the mortality information because that did not apply to me.

I was scheduled to return the next week for the Sandostatin injection. In the meantime, he did meet with the surgical team. He called to tell me that the consensus was that I was inoperable for the reasons he previously shared with me. I was disappointed with the decision. The enemy tried to sidetrack me by having me think that decision was final; I was inoperable, so I wouldn't be healed. But, I continued to trust God and believe what He said.

Scripture Confirmation:

Abraham believed the Lord, and he credited it to him as righteousness. **Genesis 15:6 NIV**

Look to the Lord and his strength; seek his face always. **1 Chronicles 16:11 NIV**

So do not fear, for I am with you; do not be dismayed, for I am your God. I will strengthen you and help you; I will uphold you with my righteous right hand. **Isaiah 41:10 NIV**

As I prayed about the results, God advised me to continue researching cancer centers that specialized in neuroendocrine cancer. The next place I found was MD Anderson Cancer Center in Houston, Texas. I called my insurance company to find out if it was in-network, although, it did not matter to me. I was going whether it was covered or not. MD Anderson Cancer Center was in-network, so I called to make an appointment. Documents were sent to me to complete so that my medical records, biopsy samples, and scans could be obtained. I was told someone would call me to schedule an appointment. Several weeks went by and no one called. I called to determine when they could see me and was told my records were still being reviewed. I felt a sense of urgency, yet felt that the staff there did not.

In the meantime, my son Jordan was also conducting research. He called me at work one day to share with me a number of innovative treatments being used at a few cancer centers across the country. We looked at MD

Anderson, which I had already contacted, Moffitt Cancer Center in Tampa, Florida, and Cancer Treatment Centers of America (CTCA).

The Cancer Treatment Centers of America website detailed a particular liver therapy that I had previously read about. I called the center to obtain additional information. Speaking with the attendant was like a breath of fresh air! The individual was so calming and knowledgeable. After learning about me and what I was dealing with, he assured me that the physicians there were aware of the latest treatments and best practices and that they would take great care of me. After he shared different treatments that may be available to me, he indicated that there was a surgeon at the Chicago location who studied under the physician who developed one procedure that I may benefit from. The procedure was the HIPEC, Hyperthermic Intraperitoneal Chemotherapy. This procedure uses a highly concentrated, heated chemotherapy that is delivered directly to the cancer cells in the abdominal area during surgery. He said if I was his sister that is the location he would recommend. I indicated my interest, and proceeded to the next step of providing my contact information for someone to call me back. Within an hour, I was contacted to select dates for my appointment. I was informed that Cancer Treatment Centers of America would fly me and a companion there for the initial medical screening and diagnosis at no cost. The Center paid for the flight and hotel stay. My husband, Gary went with me, along with my sister, Eleanor. I was told to expect to be there at least one week. Upon arrival at the airport, we were picked up in a limousine. The next day began a series of medical appointments. I was first met by a counselor who gave us an overview of the Center and what to expect during the week. I then met with the Intake Oncologist, who appeared to be a very brilliant physician. As soon as I told him the symptoms I had experienced over the years, he immediately said "Did no one check you for carcinoid or neuroendocrine cancer?" I said "no." He said those are classic symptoms. Everyone we met was extremely kind and efficient. When tests or scans were ordered, they were immediately scheduled and the results were available within hours. I was impressed with the efficiency. The staff made sure every need was attended to.

At the end of the week, I met with the oncologist I would be assigned to. He confirmed the diagnosis of neuroendocrine cancer with an unknown primary, although he suspected it was in my small intestines. He indicated that the cancer had spread to the mesenteric area, which is the area containing lymph nodes in the abdominal area. He described it as a netting like structure that holds the organs in the abdominal area. In addition, there were approximately eight tumors of varying sizes on my liver. As he looked over previous scan results to compare with those I had while there, he asked me if I had already began treatment at home through my local oncologist. I answered "no, why?" He said "because some of the tumors have begun shrinking on their own. The scans you took this week show that some tumors are now smaller than they were a month ago." Praise God!! I replied, "That's God and the power of prayer!" I begin to thank God. He was again confirming that I was healed!

The oncologist recommended that I begin treatment of 20mg of Sandostatin every four weeks. He said he would also schedule me for a surgery consult on my next visit. I received the injection after our visit. It wasn't too bad; however, after we left his office and walked to the elevator, I became somewhat heated and dizzy. After a few moments, it passed. That evening, I had an upset stomach and diarrhea.

The diarrhea continued for about a week. On day two, after returning home, I got up to go in to work. I was not feeling my best; however, I was scheduled to attend a training I had scheduled for managers. No one, other than my manager knew what I was going through at that time and I didn't want others to think I was just lying out of work.

I had just recently been moved into this position as a result of the change of the State's political administration. I was moved from an appointed position when the new Governor appointed someone else to my position. I didn't want to appear as if I was staying out of work in opposition of the job change. Gary tried to talk me into staying home, but I pressed my way to the training. That morning, I prayed and asked God to not let me experience those side effects from the future injections. Guess what, I never experienced those side effects again! Additional confirmation that God hears and answers our prayers!

Scripture Confirmation:

> *…You do not have because you do not ask God.*
> **James 4:2 NIV**

Other neuroendocrine patients I communicated with through a private Facebook group who saw other practitioners spoke of additional side effects of the injection, including a knot at the injection site, not being able to sleep on the side where they had the injection, extreme pain, not being able to walk for a few days, and others. Thank God, I never experienced any of those side effects! God kept me!

Four weeks later, on my next visit, my son Jordan met me in Chicago. He wanted an opportunity to talk with the doctors and hear firsthand what was going on. On this visit, I met with the surgeon. He stated he did not recommend surgery for me. His reason was first because the location of the primary tumor was unknown. He said doing surgery without removing the primary would likely result in it releasing more tumors after the visible tumors were removed. He said doing exploratory surgery to find the primary would possibly be too invasive. In addition, he said the location of the mesenteric tumor was too close to a major artery and there were too many tumors throughout the liver to go in and cut out. He said at that time he would not recommend it and we would see how things progressed. It sounded rational; however, I was disappointed again. As I previously indicated, I read that the best course of treatment was surgery to remove the tumors when it could be done. However, I continued to trust God!

Scripture Confirmation:

> *"For I know the plans I have for you," declares the Lord, "plans to prosper you and not to harm you, plans to give you hope and a future."*
> **Jeremiah 29:11 NIV**

God led me back to research. Although I was at one of the best cancer centers, God showed me that the surgeon was not a neuroendocrine specialist. I had heard a great deal about a neuroendocrine specialist at Vanderbilt Cancer Center in Nashville, Tennessee. I reviewed some of his online research and PowerPoint presentations from various conferences. I also found information about another renowned specialist in Louisiana.

I contacted the specialist's office at Vanderbilt Cancer Center, in Nashville, Tennessee and made an appointment. Gary and Eleanor traveled with me. Of course, this turned into a shopping trip for Eleanor and me! Everywhere we turned ladies and men were fashionably wearing cowboy boots. I liked the look, so our quest began to find the perfect pair! Of course, I found many boots that I liked. I found the prices ranged from hundreds of dollars to thousands of dollars. There were so many choices! I love quality and uniqueness; however, know that I did not spend thousands of dollars for my pair of cowboy boots.

My mornings in Nashville began with a shot of wheatgrass juice with a slice of orange. The benefits of wheatgrass include supplying the body with vitamins, boosting the immune system, and detoxifying the body. In addition, it provides a source of energy.

I met with the specialist at Vanderbilt, who reviewed my scans and medical records. He indicated that my case was classic, meaning, he sees patients regularly with the same diagnosis and tumor sites. He indicated that the tumors were indeed operable! He said he recommended that I have surgery. He further indicated that because I was doing so well, with no side effects, or symptoms that I did not have to have surgery immediately; however, he recommended that

I have surgery while I was young, and otherwise healthy. He scheduled a follow-up appointment for an MRI, I had previously only had CT Scans, but he indicated an MRI was the best scan to clearly see tumors in the liver. He also wanted me to have an Echocardiogram to check my heart because sometimes neuroendocrine tumors affect the heart. The next month, Eleanor and I returned for the additional tests. The MRI revealed about 12 spots on my liver, rather than eight. He indicated he was not concerned because I had so much healthy liver tissue. That was refreshing to hear! The Echocardiogram was fine; my heart was in great shape!

A couple of months later, during a visit to CTCA, the CT scan I had indicated growth in the size of some of the lesions in my liver. Receiving this news, I was upset. After consulting with the oncologist, he indicated that perhaps we should look at other treatments, which could include TheraSphere, a procedure where radioactive beads would be inserted intravenously to the liver to attack and destroy the blood supply to the tumors, or a chemotherapy pill. After learning of the potential side effects of both, TheraSphere beads destroying healthy liver tissue or the standard side effects of chemotherapy, I decided to take some time and pray about it. My oncologist scheduled a consultation the next day for me to speak with a radiology oncologist to review the scan and discuss TheraSphere. Once I was back in my hotel room, I sent a private message to the neuroendocrine specialist I had seen at Vanderbilt Cancer Center. He indicated that he would like to see me again and the scan that was taken. I requested an appointment because if we had to, I was going to move forth with surgery.

Reflecting on everything, I sought God and began to cry. God revealed to me that there was a measurement error and there was no new growth. He had me to review the scan results and compare to a previous scan. I did and noticed that the increase spoken of was only .5mm. At that point, I felt much better and ready to have the discussion with the radiology oncologist.

The next day, I first met with the physician assistant in the office of the radiology oncologist. I advised her that I didn't mind discussing routine information with her; however, I needed to speak with the oncologist. She understood and indicated he was doing a procedure, but she would send a message asking that he come meet with us upon completion. He did come in. Of course, one of my first questions was whether the increase shown could have been a measurement error. He said, "Let's look at your previous scans." He first looked at the MRI from Vanderbilt, and then the last two scans from CTCA. He then said, "Certainly!" He said the pictures are not clear on this last CT, which resulted in mismeasurement of some of the tumor sizes! He said "There has been no growth and you do not need TheraSphere!" Thank you Lord! God was again on point! This reassurance allowed me to again be at peace. I knew and still know that I can trust God!

Scripture Confirmation:

For the word of the LORD is right and true; he is faithful in all he does. **Psalm 33:4 NIV**

Look to the LORD and his strength; seek his

*face always. **1 Chronicles 16:11 NIV***

God will always be The Way when there seems to be no way! We have to put all of our trust in him! He is so worthy to be honored, glorified, and praised!

The news that there had been no growth was great news! When dealing with a cancer diagnosis, a report that tumors are stable is welcomed news! However, I still couldn't rest, God said I was healed, and I knew healing was on the way! I was to see the neuroendocrine specialist in four weeks. Three weeks before my appointment I received a telephone call indicating that my specialist was leaving Vanderbilt. He was unsure of when he would reestablish his practice.

I was aware that this specialist was looking to change locations, so I was not that surprised. I took solace in the fact that he had already informed me that I could take my time about deciding on surgery. When we did discuss the option of surgery, he indicated that I would have to go through two surgeries, one to remove tumors in my abdominal area, and once that healed surgery to remove the tumors in my liver. I wanted to wait for the perfect time, God's time, so I continued to pray for God's direction and favor.

CHAPTER FOUR

Following God's Advice

When the specialist I was seeing left practice, I was a bit unsure of what I would do next. Should I wait until he reestablished his practice or do I move on to another one. I again sought God.

Remember I told you about the private Facebook Page for Neuroendocrine patients and physicians? Well, I posted a question in the group inquiring about the most effective treatments for neuroendocrine tumors, specifically those with an unknown primary and metastases to the mesentery and liver. One of the responses I received was from another renowned Neuroendocrine Specialist. He indicated that he had written a Medical Journal Article on this topic. He provided me with his assistant's name and telephone number and said for me to call her and have her email me the information. He further indicated that after I read the information, if I had questions, I could contact him. He posted his personal cellphone number in the group! What specialist provides a personal cellphone number? One who really cares!

I contacted his assistant who immediately emailed me the information. After reading the material, I knew that surgery was the best option for me. I spoke with my husband, Gary and shared that I knew we had visited several doctors, seeking out treatment, but I needed to get an opinion from another Neuroendocrine Specialist. I told him about my contact with the specialist in New Orleans and indicated that I would like to go see him.

Thus far I had had two surgeons to say I was inoperable, and one who was a NET specialist say surgery was an option. I wanted another qualifying opinion. Traveling to other states, including flight expenses, hotel stays, rental car fees, and meals is expensive and my family and I had spent a great deal of money thus far. However, I was fighting to live! When fighting to live you have to declare victory and that you will give it all you have. I think of boxers and the rigorous training they endure. Even when they are tired and frustrated, they push themselves in hopes of victory! That was the mentality I had and the mentality that you must have for yourselves or in support of your loved one! Gary agreed that he was supportive and I made the appointment.

I called the office, expecting a long wait, because of this specialist's popularity. I was scheduled within a few weeks. He provided orders for me to have bloodwork done locally as well as an Octreoscan. An Octreoscan is a nuclear medicine scan that picks up traces of a radioactive compound injected intravenously and highlights any tumors found. He ordered my medical records and slides from the initial biopsy.

On September 2, 2014, my husband, Gary and my sister Eleanor, my brother-in-law, and my mother-in-law, traveled with me to New Orleans. Of course we spent that beautiful, hot day, enjoying the classic Cajun cuisine as well as sightseeing since some of them had not been to "NOLA" before.

The next morning Gary, Eleanor, and I went to my appointment. The nurse who took my vitals and history asked how I found their practice. I shared with her how I connected with this renowned oncologist via Facebook. She said to me, "honey that was God!" I considered this another "God Moment." God was again confirming that he was with me and I was following his guidance! The nurse then said to me, "These doctors are 'believers' they act and operate under the authority of God. Tell them everything they need to know and ask all questions you have. What they tell you will be accurate and the treatment they recommend will be best for you." I sat there in awe, knowing that God was using this nurse to speak to me and give me assurance.

The doctor came in and warmly greeted us. He pulled up my medical records and scans and discussed them with us. He indicated that his mother was diagnosed with the same type cancer and ironically, it was in the same areas as he noted in my body. He said, "We took excellent care of her and we will do the same for you!" Yes, God, thank you! That was another "God Moment!"

The oncologist drew a diagram of the tumors in my body. He described my situation as the "Cinderella Story." He explained I was at the ball, dancing with my handsome prince. Gary interjected and said, "That has to be me!" Doc said, "I would hope so!" He said the current treatment I was receiving, the Sandostatin injections were stopping the clock. However, without further interjection, the clock would strike midnight. However, if I had surgery, the clock would be set back to the time where the ball begin, the point where there were no tumors, or at least fewer, which would give us more time dancing at the ball.

He indicated that the surgery would be extensive. It was expected to take eight to ten hours and I would be in the hospital for about ten days. Because the surgery was so long, he indicated, he would team with a partner. He said, "You don't want me operating on you if I am tired or hungry! With a partner, I can stop and go eat, and he can continue." That made perfect sense and I was grateful for his wisdom. He said he wanted me to meet his partner and make sure I was comfortable with him as well.

His partner, who is just as brilliant and humorous, came in. He explained what would take place during surgery. He said, "When operating, I listen to God; I go where he tells me to go, and I stop when he tells me to stop!" By now, I am about to leap out of the chair!

He said, so when do you want to have surgery? I thought for a moment, and said, "late December or sometime in January." He said "Why do you need to wait that long?" I said, "Because I want to get through the holidays feeling good." He then said, "If you would have surgery next month, you will be healed by the holidays!" I remembered what the nurse said. If he was recommending surgery sooner, that was what I should do. I indicated I would move forth and asked what dates in October were available. We scheduled October 22, 2014. We all left feeling confident in the decision. We spent the remainder of the day enjoying more great Cajun cuisine.

CHAPTER FIVE

Giving God the Glory

A week later, I received a call from the surgeon's office; the nurse put him on the line. He indicated he had just received a call to speak at a National conference about neuroendocrine cancer and the innovative surgical procedures used in his practice. He said, "I would have to fly out the day after your surgery but I would not want to leave you like that. I don't anticipate any complications, but I would want to be around for you." He asked if I would mind moving surgery up a week or back a week so that he could speak at the conference. I told him I appreciated his concern and it would be no problem. Surgery was rescheduled for October 29, 2014.

I spent the week before surgery in Orlando with Jordan and Meagan. Jordan flew with me from Orlando to New Orleans on October 27th. Gary met us later that evening. The next day, my sisters, Patricia, Eleanor, and Carolyn arrived. I was so blessed to have so much support from my family during this time! This brought me peace and comfort knowing that God was with me, and so was my family.

On the morning of October 28th we all met at one of my

favorite breakfast spots, IHOP. Breakfast was delicious. I couldn't eat it all, but knew it would be my last solid meal of the day. I couldn't eat anything solid after 10:00 a.m. Once I completed the pre-op exams and consultations, we went to the hotel where my sisters were staying. Their suite was packed with grocery and snacks, all of the things I like, but couldn't have. They did have broth and popsicles for me.

Later, they decided they were going out to eat, I think it was Gary who wanted to have Louisiana fried chicken. I decided I would remain at the hotel until they returned. That would have been torture, sitting there smelling delicious food and not being able to have any. I lay on the couch drinking chicken broth and eating popsicles until they returned.

We all stayed together until about 10:00 pm. Gary, Jordan, and I returned to the Hope Lodge, where we were staying. The Hope Lodge is a beautiful facility built by the American Cancer Society. There are locations across the country that provide complimentary accommodations for cancer patients and a companion when the patients are having medical treatment. The accommodations in New Orleans are very nice. It is a hotel-like facility with a kitchen, dining room, and laundry rooms on each floor for guests.

On the morning of surgery, October 29, 2014, I awoke, prayed, and showered, in preparation for surgery. Gary picked up my sisters and we all left for the hospital. In the pre-op room, we prayed, and then all of the usual joking and laughter begin. Shortly thereafter, the team begin coming through to talk to me, nurses, anesthesiologists, and of course, my surgeon. He said, "God's got this!" That's all I needed to hear! Next came the intravenous injections, we all exchanged kisses, I love you, and I was rolled down the hall.

I woke up in ICU with my son, Jordan rubbing my hand. He asked how I felt. He told me my response was "Like I've been hit by a Mack truck!" Gary was in the room also. I recall Jordan saying "it's gone Mommy! You don't have cancer anymore! I said "To God be the glory." I still tear up and get chills when I think about that! We serve an awesome God who is faithful and his word is true!

Scripture Confirmation:

> *So is my word that goes out from my mouth: it will not return to me empty, but will accomplish what I desire and achieve the purpose for which I sent it.* **Isaiah 55:11 NIV**

> *Know therefore that the Lord your God is God; he is the faithful God, keeping his covenant of love to a thousand generations of those who love him and keep his commandments.* **Deuteronomy 7:9 NIV**

My sisters came in the room, tears of joy were flowing! They too were so elated at the mighty work God had done! My dad was on the phone, he said he had been anxiously waiting for the call to say I was fine. It was a joyous and tearful day. Of course, I was sleeping and waking all day. Later my surgeon came by. He gave all the credit to God. He said the surgery only took five hours; he found and removed the primary tumor and he removed all that he could see. As a bonus, he said he removed my ovaries, since I wouldn't be needing those! Well, I was drowsy, but I knew what that meant!

I had the best ICU nurse ever! He took great care of me and my every need. He made me feel as though I was his only patient. He even allowed Gary to spend the night in ICU with me. He and Jordan bonded and when I would wake the three of them would be talking and laughing. He and Jordan still communicate.

The second day, the nurse came in and said, we're kicking you out and sending you to your own room since you're doing so well! Originally, I was told I would be in ICU about three days. Later she came back in and said, you are getting the best room on the floor! That was God's favor! She said you have so much support; we are giving you the biggest room with a nice view, of course!

My surgeon came by to check on me each day, on the first day after being moved to my private room, he came by. He discussed the surgery with me. I said, "Doc, you are the man of the hour." His reply was, "No, God is the man of the hour!" That's my kind of physician, one who gives God the glory and recognizes that God is the Master Physician!" On the fourth day of my hospital stay, my surgeon came in and said, "It's time for you to go home!" He said, you're doing great and I don't want you just lying around here and get some kind of infection. Go home where you can rest, relax, and completely heal. Gary arranged our flights and we flew out the next day.

The next two weeks, I spent on the coast, at my father's home, where he, Gary, and my sisters took excellent care of me. I experienced very little pain and discomfort during the entire healing process! I give all glory to God for keeping me.

Scripture Confirmation:

The Lord watches over you—the Lord is your shade at your right hand. **Psalm 121:5 NIV**

Just as my surgeon promised me, I was well during the holidays. I spent Thanksgiving in Wilmington, North Carolina with my family. Though I didn't eat much, I was able to enjoy some of what I wanted, but most importantly, I was well and able to enjoy spending time with my family. We spent Christmas day at our home. I prepared dinner, then we left again, the following day to travel to Wilmington to be with my extended family. Each day, I became stronger and stronger. I even begin walking for exercise. I lost about 15 pounds during this time; however, that was a good thing! I didn't miss them!

During my recovery period, I watched my church services online. I thank God for my church's livestream, Wake Chapel Church, Raleigh, North Carolina. **www. wakechapel.org**

Pastor Wilkins' anointing seemed to penetrate the computer screen. Even at home, I was blessed!

By the end of December, I was becoming restless being at home. I did get adequate rest, but I was ready to get back to a more regular routine. I went back to work on January 12, 2015. God restored me!

CHAPTER SIX

You Don't Look Sick

Throughout this journey, so frequently I would hear the words, "you don't look sick." Thanks be to God, they were right. As I reflected on those words, I would think, and I don't feel sick. God is keeping me and His power will keep you also, be encouraged!

We see hundreds of people on any given day. Some may be well dressed, some may be dressed casually, some may be smiling, and some may not. We don't know what they may be dealing with beneath the pretty clothes or smiling faces. No I don't look sick. I haven't looked sick for the four years this disease has quietly invaded my cells. God is keeping me and I am grateful!

Get up every morning, whether you feel like it or not and be determined that you will have a good day. Get dressed, even dressed up, makeup and all! You'll be surprised what a difference it makes in the way you feel.

For every doctor's appointment, I was well dressed and fully made up with jewelry and accessories. I would often look around at some others and think to myself, they're probably wondering "where does she think she's going."

When facing trials, it is imperative that no matter what, you have the right attitude. The right attitude is one of strong faith, keeping your head up and smiling through the trial, knowing that you are not alone. No one was able to look at me and tell that I was going through anything. I was standing on the Word and promises of God, just as you must do!

Is your hurt or pain greater than the Power of God? No! Concentrate on God; He will bring the high mountains down!

The brain has a huge impact over our bodies. Use you time thinking positive thoughts and saying positive affirmations.

Scripture Confirmation:

> *For as he thinks in his heart, so is he….* ***Proverbs 23:7 NKJV***

Always be aware of what is going on in your mind, you have control over your thoughts. Positive thoughts, prayer, and meditations are hard to measure scientifically; however, studies have shown that these strategies can affect how we heal or deal with pain and difficulty.

Throughout my journey, I prayed, meditated on scriptures, and listened to songs of healing daily. I had a "healing playlist" on my iPhone. Those songs became a part of my soul as did the scriptures I read or listened to daily. It is good to read the Word of God aloud as well as silently. I also listened to healing scriptures while driving, or cooking.

Scripture Confirmation:

Consequently, faith comes from hearing the message, and the message is heard through the Word about Christ. **Romans 10:17 NIV**

Relax, relax, relax, and avoid stress. Stress kills and fosters many maladies in our bodies. Relax by reading, journaling, exercising, or listening to music. Also, take personal time for yourself. I have a membership at Massage Envy. Monthly, I treat myself to a massage or two! Another beneficial practice for relaxation includes the use of essential oils. There are essential oils for relaxing, meditating, and healing of your body and mind. I was surprised at the true benefits I experienced from the use of essential oils. My particular favorites include Frankincense for healing and meditation, Lavender for calming and relaxation, Peppermint for uplifting and easing stomach issues, Orange for uplifting my spirits, and Eucalyptus to cleanse the environment and boost my immune system. There are many more. I diffuse the scents throughout my home, automobile, and office. I also use them in my shower or bath. Aromatherapy can play a major role in maintaining a healthy attitude.

CHAPTER SEVEN

Caregivers... The Faith of Those around You

There is a story in the Bible about a man who was paralyzed. He heard Jesus would be in town teaching and desired to go. He was bed ridden. He had four friends who carried him on his bed to the place where Jesus was. The crowd was so enormous that they went on the roof, removed some of the roof, and lowered their friend through the roof to be healed by Jesus. Jesus saw the faith of his friends and healed the paralytic man, both physically and spiritually. **(Luke 5:17-26)** Because of the faith of his friends, he was healed!

This story is the perfect example of the importance of having people around you who sincerely care about your well-being, will carry you, pray for you, travel to medical appointments with you, love you, and most importantly have faith!

I am blessed to have had family members travel with me to medical appointments in state and out of state. They were always there for me to address any need I had.

Your wellbeing can greatly be impacted by the thoughts, words, and actions of those around you. You know who those people are in your life. If you are not sure, pray and ask God to give you discernment to know who they are. When God shows you, those are the people you want around you and praying for you! There may be times when you don't know what else to pray for or you may be in a state where you can't pray, it is important to know that there are others who will keep the prayers going on your behalf.

Among those praying for you should be the Elders of the Church as set out in the Bible.

Scripture Confirmation:

> *Is any among you sick? Let them call the elders of the church to pray over them and anoint them with oil in the name of the Lord. And the prayer offered in faith will make the sick person well; the Lord will raise them up. If they have sinned, they will be forgiven.* **James 5:14-15 NIV**

I thank God for my family members, my Pastor and first lady, church Elders, Deacons, Deacon Wives, and dear friends who were there for me.

Some prayed, some visited, some sent cards, some sent flowers and fruit arrangements, some purchased and delivered meals, and some called or texted. Whatever the deed, I will be forever grateful!

Caregivers should not be neglected or taken advantage of, they also need some downtime. It can be exhausting, giving your all, taking care of others. Be sure to show your appreciation for your caregivers. Pray for them and their strength in addition to praying for any needs they may have.

CHAPTER EIGHT

Resources

Having a diagnosis of cancer or other chronic illness can be very expensive; especially being faced with a rare cancer diagnosis as I was. Because there were no local specialists, I had to travel to three different states for opinions and treatment. For me one treatment visit could amount to over $28, 000.00 per month. The injection alone was $15,000.00. I thank God for good health insurance! Although I have good health insurance, there are still out of pocket expenses such as copays, airline ticket costs, rental car costs, hotel costs, costs for medicine and supplements, and meals. All of these costs are in addition to ongoing monthly expenses prior to the diagnosis.

Many people diagnosed with cancer or other chronic illnesses have difficulty with all of the added financial obligations, believe me, I know. On this journey, I met many people and heard many stories. Through my research for myself and others, I found several resources that may be beneficial.

Included in these references are a compilation of healing scriptures as well as my iPhone Healing Playlist. May these all be a blessing to you.

One of the resources is a 501(c)(3) where I serve as a proud board member. The Sisters Inspiring Sisters. (SISI) Inc. www.thesisi.org

Helpful Websites

American Society of Clinical Oncology Resources
www.cancer.net

American Cancer Society
www.cancer.org

Association of Cancer Online Resources (ACOR)
www.acor.org

National Coalition for Cancer Survivorship
www.canceradvocacy.org

The Carcinoid Foundation
www.carcinoid.org

Financial and Pharmaceutical Resources
www.patientresource.com/financial_resources.aspx

General and Financial Resources
www.managecancer.org

Transportation Assistance and Awareness
www.thesisi.org

Cancer Treatment Centers of America
www.cancercenter.com

Ochsner Neuroendocrine Tumor Clinic
**www.ochsner.org/services/
neuroendocrine-tumor-program**

Support and Online Communities
https://reimagine.me

Prayer

Prayer@wakechapel.org

<u>Some of My Favorite Healing Scriptures</u>

Dear friend, I hope all is well with you and that you are as healthy in body as you are strong in spirit. **3 John 1:2 NLT**

"For I know the plans I have for you," says the Lord, "They are plans for good and not for disaster, to give you a future and a hope." Jeremiah **29:11 NLT**

Let us then approach God's throne of grace with confidence, so that we may receive mercy and find grace to help us in our time of need. **Hebrews 4:16 NIV**

Trust in the Lord with all your heart and lean not on your own understanding; in all your ways submit to him, and he will make your paths straight. **Proverbs 3:5, 6 NIV**

But blessed is the one who trust in the Lord, whose confidence is in him. They will be like a tree planted by the water that sends out its roots by the stream. It does not fear when heat comes; its leaves are always green. It has no worries in a year of drought and never fails to bear fruit. **Jeremiah 17: 7-8 NIV**

For the Lord will be at your side and will keep your foot from being snared. **Proverbs 3:26 NIV**

Abraham believed the Lord, and he credited it to

him as righteousness. **Genesis 15:6 NIV**

Look to the Lord and his strength; seek his face always. **1 Chronicles 16:11 NIV**

So do not fear, for I am with you; do not be dismayed, for I am your God. I will strengthen you and help you; I will uphold you with my righteous right hand. **Isaiah 41:10 NIV**

…You do not have because you do not ask God. **James 4:2 NIV**

For the word of the LORD is right and true; he is faithful in all he does. **Psalm 33:4 NIV**

Look to the LORD and his strength; seek his face always. **1 Chronicles 16:11 NIV**

For as he thinks in his heart, so is he…. **Proverbs 23:7 NKJV**

Consequently, faith comes from hearing the message, and the message is heard through the Word about Christ. Romans **10:17 NIV**

So is my word that goes out from my mouth: it will not return to me empty, but will accomplish what I desire and achieve the purpose for which I sent it. **Isaiah 55:11 NIV**

Know therefore that the Lord your God is God; he is the faithful God, keeping his covenant of love to a thousand generations of those who love him and keep his commandments. **Deuteronomy 7:9 NIV**

The Lord watches over you—the Lord is your shade at your right hand. **Psalm 121:5 NIV**

Is any among you sick? Let them call the elders of the church to pray over them and anoint them with oil in the name of the Lord. And the prayer offered in faith will make the sick person well; the Lord will raise them up. If they have sinned, they will be forgiven. **James 5:14-15 NIV**

<u>Songs from My iPhone Healing Playlist</u>

I Am the God That Healeth Thee, Don Moen, Give Thanks

I'm Healed (Live) Victory In Praise Music and Arts Seminar, Any Day

Standing In the Need, The New Life Community Choir, The Essential John P. Keep

The Lord Is Able, John P. Kee, Show Up

Healed, Donald Lawrence, Speak Life

Praise Jehovah, Beverly Crawford, Live from Los Angeles

Holy, Holy, Holy, CeCe Winans & Pure Worship

God Favored Me, Hezekiah Walker, Souled Out

Grateful, Hezekiah Walker & The Love Fellowship Choir

God Blocked It (Live), Kurt Carr, The Very Best of Kurt Carr & The Kurt Carr Singers

He Has His Hands On You, Marvin Sapp, Here I Am

It Ain't Over, Marlette Brown Clark, The Dream

Healing, Richard Smallwood (with Vision) (Live In Detroit)

I'm Still Standing, Bishop Paul S. Morton, Still Standing

Be Blessed, Bishop Paul S. Morton, Still Standing

www.ingramcontent.com/pod-product-compliance
Lightning Source LLC
Chambersburg PA
CBHW051416250726
48655CB00003B/1076